Stop Allergies
From Ruining Your Life

D0887830

Stop Allergies
From Ruining Your Life
The Easy Way

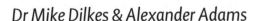

Dr Mike Dilkes & Alexander Adams

First published in Great Britain in 2018 by Orion Spring
an imprint of The Orion Publishing Group Ltd
Carmelite House, 50 Victoria Embankment
London ES4Y 0DZ

An Hachette UK Company

1 3 5 7 9 10 8 6 4 2

Every effort has been made to ensure that the information in the book is
accurate. The information in this book may not be applicable in each individual
case so it is advised that professional medical advice is obtained for specific
health matters and before changing any medication or dosage. Neither the
publisher nor author accepts any legal responsibility for any personal injury
or other damage or loss arising from the use of the information in this book.
In addition if you are concerned about your diet or exercise regime and wish
to change them, you should consult a health practitioner first.

A CIP catalogue record for this book is
available from the British Library.

ISBN (Trade Paperback): 978 1 8418 8273 4
ISBN (ebook): 978 1 8418 8274 1

Printed in Great Britain by CPI Group (UK) Ltd, Croydon, CR0 4YY

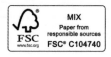

www.orionbooks.co.uk

ORION
SPRING

Contents

Introduction

Allergies have unfortunately become a mainstay of daily life for millions of people worldwide, whether it be the seasonal congestion and flu-like symptoms of the hay fever patient, paranoia over the contents of everyday foods in the food allergy sufferer or the endless daily routine of irritated, uncomfortable-feeling skin and sleepless nights endured by the eczema patient. Conditions like this can be maddening and seem endless. Ironically (given their prevalence) allergies can leave people feeling isolated and lonely. Putting a stop to the plight of allergy is long overdue.

The aim of this book is to level a heavily overcrowded playing field and make clear sense of a problem that has become unnecessarily complex. We will outline the three core areas that trigger an allergic response and will provide a universal go-to – enabling the reader to understand the problem, dispel the myth and give sound proven advice on prevention as well as proactive remedies to ease outbreaks.

Allergy is a problem. The numbers of those affected are at historic highs – with everything from beaver top hats to red velvet cupcakes being unearthed as triggers.[1] The good news is that allergy is not a problem we can't prevent and it is most certainly a problem that can be effectively remedied.

The real issue here relates much more to the fact that until now, no one could tell you exactly what allergy is. Getting to grips with all the available information can seem like an impossible task. Indeed, the sheer volume of online search results when simply looking for basic answers to very basic questions is astonishing. Equally surprising is the number of differing opinions and infinite possible causes.

Allergy originated in animals as a means of expelling noxious or potentially dangerous substances such as poisons, toxins and parasites within seconds of being exposed to them – much faster than a traditional immune reaction, although the underlying mechanism is the same. And that is because these toxins can be lethal within minutes – so there is not enough time for a traditional immune response, and parasites, once embedded, can be hard to recognise – not least since they have inbuilt mechanisms to trick the body's immune response. In a sense then, the fact that people do have an allergic response is a good thing. The body is functioning as intended and is primed to pinpoint the difference between a benefit and a poison. However, the conditions we categorise as allergic reactions are a misfiring of this natural vetting process, the problem being that the allergy sufferer cannot always distinguish properly between a benefit and a poison. Non-threatening substances such as grass pollen can therefore invoke the same expulsion reaction as a poison would.

It is understandable to think that the logical people to ask for clear advice about these abnormal allergic responses are the experts: the pharmaceutical companies, academic institutions and medical practitioners whose recommendations and prescriptions are surely evidence of a true grasp of the problem at hand. In reality, the problem of clarity around allergy is a direct result of the medical community's own ongoing saga in defining it – an issue that has been a constant theme since the 1800s. And to this day, the term 'allergy' fails to have a well-defined meaning, even among healthcare professionals.[2]

Part of the challenge is, as always, human nature and our tendency to be drawn towards, and then normalise, the most extreme of scenarios. We are far more intrigued by *My Girl*-style deaths via bee sting-induced anaphylaxis, and ways of preventing those than we are about really understanding the simple solutions to the common conditions that we are likely to suffer from. Regardless, the narrative around allergic reactions unrelentingly focuses on these rare cases.

The actual incidence of death from anaphylaxis in a country of 65 million people, such as the UK, is around 30 cases per year.[3] These are mainly due to insect stings or drug reactions. Food allergy deaths are very rare, 6 per year in the UK. Admissions from anaphylaxis or suspected anaphylaxis have shot up, but death from such an admission is also rare – only 1 in 50 of these patients have a cardiopulmonary arrest. So, awareness is increasing, and treatment is very effective.*

It is not the purpose of this book to continue this trend and give more airtime to the tiny fraction of causes that still dominate the allergy conversation. It is essential to focus instead on the majority of cases of protracted everyday symptoms that cause daily discomfort and misery to approaching 50 per cent of the world's population.[4] But with clarity of definition and short, easy to follow regimes, sufferers can experience a dramatic improvement in their quality of life.

---

* Interestingly, there are no similar campaigns regarding equally dangerous pursuits, such as choking on food (220 deaths in the UK per year) or lying under a coconut tree (150 deaths per year worldwide).

Self-Diagnosis and Silent Suffering?

The murkiness involved in finding simple solutions to common problems is not helped by a significant trend in patients/sufferers taking their health into their own hands and entering the realm of self-diagnosis. Positively changing one's habits is, of course, not something to be scoffed at and we would hope that this move to take due diligence in personal research would make the whole process, from diagnosis to cure, vastly more streamlined. Yet this is far from the case. Endless choice is the fairy tale of consumerism and you would think that all of the medical advice available online would enhance our choice of diagnosis and treatment. However, the key difference with allergy is that when we think about consumer or buying choices, the main objective for companies and brands is to make sense of all the noise on your behalf so that you, the consumer, err on the side of their product. They have funnelled an infinite landscape of choice into a handful of simple products that leave the consumer happy with the outcome and likely to return.

When we look at medical advice through the same 'buying' lens, however, the exact opposite is true. The noise is ever increasing and making matters far more confusing and unsatisfying. The American psychologist Barry Schwartz has famously defined this as the 'Paradox of Choice', where we are bombarded with so many options that we retreat from a definitive medical diagnosis and in some cases never make one at all.

The subsequent rise in self-diagnosis is the stem of many issues when it comes to basic health, especially allergy. Being on the same side of the table as your medical professional is essential – therefore the benefit of a clean slate when it comes to check-ups cannot be stressed enough. Research conducted by the patient prior to their appointment can drive the conversation and misdirect the discussion away from more likely root causes. As we will discuss throughout this book, an open and honest dialogue with your GP is essential to ensure a truly accurate appraisal of your health. Be a team – this saves you the anguish of untold possible search engine results and more importantly the swathe of often quite unnecessary medical testing that follows, along with being labelled allergic via your GP notes, for the rest of your life, when this may not be the case at all.

Fear of Allergens

More than anything, it is the anxiety and abject fear of allergy that can consume someone's day – an anxiety that can create its own symptoms. For instance, if you have had an experience of, or have a general fear of, reacting to something you have eaten then you are likely worrying about a host of gastrointestinal problems such as bloating, nausea, abdominal pain and diarrhoea. An even more pervasive concern is the feeling that your throat is getting tight, even closing up, and that you have a difficulty in breathing.[5] This fear is totally understandable and you might be comforted to know that less than 0.0000001 per cent of the world's population actually suffers from extreme reactions to food. Ironically, however, just the abject anxiety and fear of an allergic reaction can induce allergy-like physical symptoms. So if you worry about a foodstuff giving you an upset stomach at the worst possible time, such as at an exam or job interview, that worry can actually bring about that exact outcome. Equally, if they have read about the rise in peanut-related deaths and proceed to eat peanuts it is common for people to feel the sensation of their throat closing up, a seeming inability to breathe properly or spells of dizziness – otherwise called panic.

Interestingly, we see that exactly the same is true in those people who worry about touching certain metals, fibres or liquids, etc. The thought of breaking out in unsightly blotches, rashes and burns is by definition an uncomfortable one. But once again we see that just the stress response can bring about physical reactions – such as outbreaks of shingles.

Fear and anxiety on the face of it are tough to treat but in reality they are simply evidence of a lack of understanding. If you are lost in the woods without even basic survival training then the prospect of being exposed to the elements night after night is impossible to come to terms with. But as is often the case, once we are equipped with some clear and easy to apply insights the unknown quickly changes into something predictable and manageable.

Taking Back Control

The real outcome here is that if we indulge too heavily in the search engine and tabloid conversations surrounding allergy we will ultimately arrive at a point where we have lowered the standard of what we call advice. The aim of this book is to break down the science into a set of simple rules to help you help yourself.

In the chapters that follow we will give a jargon-free analysis of three core areas:

- *Inhaled* allergies
- *Ingested* allergies
- *Contact* allergies

So that we can properly discuss allergy, we first need to shed light on a much under-publicised distinction: the difference between allergic reactions and intolerance.

1.

Allergic Reactions vs Intolerance

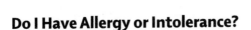

Do I Have Allergy or Intolerance?

Allergy and intolerance are often confused, and since their treatments are very different, it is important to know. The best way to distinguish between a true allergic reaction and an intolerance is through the lens of one of the most commonly discussed topics: milk, or rather one of its components, lactose. There is a serious danger in lack of understanding and paranoia, especially when it comes to children in this relatively common problem. It is completely understandable, so don't worry. By the end of this chapter you will be much clearer about the true dangers that face you and your family, which will prevent those all too frequent emergency room visits.

So let's make this clear.

Milk allergy (or indeed any allergy) describes a response from the body's immune system. This response is very rare as it signals a release of histamines in reaction to something usually harmless in the body.[6] The reaction can be rapid and potentially extremely serious if not addressed immediately. Given that less than 1 per cent of people undergo testing, if you are one of the incredibly rare few that know you have this type of immune response it is essential that you understand the real symptoms – and the means of prevention and remedy outlined below.

Making Sense of the Myth

Allergy is not the same as intolerance. Or in this case, milk allergy is not the same as milk sensitivity (lactose intolerance). Milk, or lactose, intolerance simply describes one's inability to digest the sugars that are found in most dairy products. It is important to prevent the term 'allergic' from becoming a catch-all way of describing any number of sensitivities, intolerances and (all too often) dislikes. It may surprise you that only 1–2 per cent of people actually have food allergies[7] – and yet it is assumed that vast swathes of the population are allergy prone, with new triggers discovered and publicised in the national press on a near daily basis. Most people are in reality sensitive, intolerant or they just don't like certain foods.

The aim here is to standardise the ever-growing glossary of available terms in this area. We have outlined the key distinctions between allergy and intolerance at a usefully high level. We must now take the time to dig far deeper into the biological mechanics of an allergic reaction to truly understand and appreciate this complex medical issue.

In Summary

Allergy is an unhelpfully loaded term. A quick look into the difference between an allergic reaction and an intolerance begins the process of becoming aware that in reality you and your family almost certainly suffer from the latter, as it is much more common. While the symptoms of intolerance are serious, by understanding that they are not the danger they are assumed to be we pave the way for a calm and collected approach.

2.

Allergic Reactions

What is Allergy?

Meet Callum, who is enjoying a midsummer stroll while returning from a picnic in the countryside with his friends. The air is filled with pollen from the surrounding trees and starts to cause Callum an allergic reaction – sneezing, itching, running nose and blockage – hay fever. An allergic response of this kind occurs because Callum's immune system reacts abnormally to a common substance in the environment – in this case tree pollen. Allergens such as pollen cause changes in the body that may range from mild to severe.[8] A true allergic reaction is when an antibody binds with an antigen and causes the leakage of special cells – known as basophils or mast cells (they are the same) – in the body. An antibody is a defensive protein made by the body, which mops up unwanted invaders – like viruses, bacteria, parasites, poisons, toxins, etc. The more medical term for antibody is 'immunoglobulin'.

When you first become allergic, it's because your DNA has created white blood cells called presenter cells (also known as T lymphocytes) that bind with an antigen. Simply put, an antigen is any foreign body that sparks an immune response. These presenter cells are the first line of defence as they sit in the lining of the body's outside surfaces – the nose, the lungs, the skin, the gut, etc. The allergic process repeats every time Callum encounters this pollen because the presenter cells in his nose (or any other outside surface) interact with more white blood cells, called memory cells, which in turn stimulate the formation of plasma cells, which release the antibodies (immunoglobulins) that react with the original pollen. So once the memory cells have been primed in the initial exposure via the presenter cells, the process is automatic – and often lifelong.

The evolution from presenter cell to plasma cell is as fascinating as it is essential, since it is the plasma cells that produce immunoglobulins. Also known as antibodies, immunoglobulins act as a critical part of the immune response involved in fighting infection and causing allergy. What's clever about them is that they are able to recognise specific threats and combat them in isolation. Much like choosing the right size Allen key for the job, immunoglobulins (Igs), or antibodies, come in varying classes, each designed to complete a specific task.* In the case of allergy, it is Immunoglobulin E that interacts with the pollen (the antigen) and causes mast cell degranulation and release of local inflammatory agents, like histamine.

The release of these inflammatory substances causes the changes in the body that we know as allergy and shows us that Callum has had a classic reaction to tree pollen. Along with histamine, other

---

* The toolbox looks like this:

- Immunoglobulin A (IgA): Targets mucosal membranes
- IgD: Function unknown; seems to aid IgM
- IgE: Fights parasites and noxious substances, causes allergy
- IgG: Combats pathogens, viruses and bacteria
- IgM: Early recognition of pathogens and activates IgG production

inflammatory mediators include leukotrienes and cytokines. They cause symptoms as described by Callum's experience but also a host of others depending on where they are released.

- **In the nose**
  Sneezing
  Running
  Blockage
  Itching

- **In the lungs**
  Mucus production
  Cough
  Contraction of the small tubes of the lungs – wheeze

- **In the skin**
  Itching
  Redness
  Lumps (weals or urticaria)

- **In the gut**
  Diarrhoea
  Mucus production
  Spasm (pain)
  Malabsorption (possibly)
  Vomiting

- **In the eyes**
  Itching
  Running
  Swelling

These symptoms are all part of an expulsion reaction, from runny eyes to diarrhoea, coughing and sneezing – i.e. find the problem and get it out as quickly as possible. As previously discussed, allergy originated as a protective mechanism to expel noxious or potentially dangerous substances within seconds of being exposed to them, for obvious reasons. It works much faster than a traditional virus-type immune reaction, which may take days.

How Does It Work?

It's all about the immune response. Think about the measles vaccination. You need to trick the body into thinking you have got measles, so the body makes antibodies to it – when the real measles virus then comes along it is easily defeated without illness.

Imagine the body as consisting of a series of doors that each correspond to a different virus. When you are well, each of these doors is shut. However, if you are attacked by a virus the corresponding door will swing open, letting the virus in and causing you to become very ill. What happens when you have a vaccine is that the door is opened for that virus a very small amount (therefore making you a little bit ill) but crucially, the door is thereafter permanently locked. When that virus next comes knocking, the door won't open, and you'll stay well.

The difficult with allergy is that, unlike immunisation, we can't keep the body's corresponding door permanently shut. With the help of medicine, we can close the door once it's been breached but we can't prevent an allergy from opening that door again (and again!). Instead we have to play a cat-and-mouse game of avoidance and treatment.

It's therefore extremely important that the IgE antibody response has such an immediate effect – we sneeze, cough or have diarrhoea very quickly after exposure to the problem so if it's a bug or a parasite it doesn't have enough time to burrow into the body or be absorbed before it is expelled. The same is true with the skin, where intense local reactions (called urticaria) cause the immediate expulsion of whatever is trying to get in. This remarkable defence mechanism of the body's gives us an immediate barrier of protection to outside elements (e.g. grass pollen) that we might be allergic to.

When Allergies Become Deadly

Unfortunately, this hypersensitivity reaction, created to help us, has in the end mainly served us badly, and sometimes fatally in the case of anaphylaxis.

Anaphylaxis

Anaphylaxis induces fear in the eyes of the allergy sufferer, and with good reason. It occurs when there is a massive allergic response to exposure with an allergen (antigen). Huge amounts of histamine release occur, causing swelling of the face, especially the lips and eyes, hives (a lumpy rash all over the body), wheeze and collapse. Sometimes death results, via asphyxiation (can't breathe) and a catastrophic drop in blood pressure. It occurs because particular antigens have an increased mast cell degranulation potential – for example, drugs such as penicillin, bee/wasp stings, peanuts, tree nuts, fish, milk, eggs, some fruits and shellfish. However, most other inhaled or food allergies don't.

That's what is strange about allergy and anaphylaxis – the most common allergens, such as house dust mite and tree/grass pollens, are not associated with anaphylaxis at all. It is only food, drug and wasp/bee sting allergies that cause anaphylaxis.

Now that we have a better understanding of what allergic and intolerant reactions are, it is time to uncover exactly how they apply to you.

In Summary

When an allergic reaction occurs, complex mechanisms are at work. Our body is on high alert to protect healthy function and will stop at nothing to prevent noxious substances from harming it. A malfunction in certain individuals means that an exaggerated form of this protection actually works against the impulse to protect and instead ushers in a host of symptoms that impair, irritate and cause great discomfort.

3.

Inhaled Allergies

The Air We Breathe

Inhaled or airborne allergies are by far the most common in provoking reactions from sufferers. Unlike ingested or contact allergies, where in a sense one needs to go out of one's way to encounter allergens, the act of simply breathing is far more difficult to avoid. And, as many hay fever sufferers will attest, a secondary entry point for airborne dangers is the eyes.

A Common Condition with Common Triggers

Inhaled allergies are quite common – statistics suggest that in America alone nearly 35 million people suffer from upper respiratory tract allergic symptoms. These are symptoms which reside in the major passages and structures of the respiratory system; namely the nostrils, nasal cavity, mouth, throat and voice box. These serve as the primary entry points for inhaled allergens.[9]

Triggers

When we talk about inhaled allergies we tend to describe triggers that arise from four key areas:

- Pollens
- House dust mite
- Mould spores
- Animals (typically fur or dander)

In those who are not allergic, the body simply dispatches any detected unwanted item out from whence it came with a short sharp cough or sneeze, a watering of the eyes or rapid blinking. Alternatively, it can draw it down through the throat via the mucus in the nasal passage, where it will be swallowed, digested and forgotten.

The story for an inhaled allergy sufferer is much more protracted, as histamine release triggers the onset of nasal passage swelling, blockage, running, sneezing, itching and irritation. Further down in the lungs, small airway contraction, mucus production and coughing are the results.

Is it a Cold or is it an Allergy?

Trying to determine if your symptoms are evidence of an onset of allergy or simply just a common cold is often a big part of the problem. Medical issues share many symptoms and cause great concern when the sufferer begins the process of self-diagnosis. The table below will help highlight the nuances of allergy versus a cold and help you take valuable information to your GP for a proper diagnosis:

Symptoms	Cold	Airborne Allergy
Cough	Common	Sometimes
General Aches, Pains	Common	Never
Fatigue, Weakness	Sometimes	Sometimes
Itchy Eyes	Never	Common
Sneezing	Usual	Usual
Sore Throat	Common	Sometimes
Runny Nose	Common	Common
Stuffy Nose	Common	Common
Fever	Common	Never
Duration	3 to 7 days	Weeks (for example, 6 weeks for ragweed or grass pollen seasons)

Eyes

Allergic conjunctivitis or 'pink eye' is well known to hay fever sufferers. The conjunctiva is the outer lining of the eye, the surface most exposed to the outer world. Mast cells are spread throughout the conjunctiva. These cells lie in wait for an antigen to come into contact with the area they protect and then grab hold with the aid of a specific antibody. Now that the cell has trapped the offending particle it must prevent it from causing harm, and then expel it – namely, initiate histamine release to isolate the threat. For example, a healthy outer lining to the eye is bright white with no signs of inflammation or redness. If, however, a person who reacts to chlorine has been swimming and the irritant has come into contact with the eye the exact opposite is true. We will see red inflamed eyes which will cause huge discomfort, itching and intermittent blinking. Imagine the feeling of having an eyelash in your eye – but in this instance the pain will not stop once the lash is removed. Allergy sufferers react in the same way to a host of irritants – many of which are tough to avoid, such as pollen or dust. Taken to extremes, allergic conjunctivitis causes itchy, watering eyes and often creates pools of pus which stick to the eyelashes. Very much like allergic nose disease, allergic conjunctivitis can be seasonal, when it is caused by tree/grass pollens or moulds, or it can be perennial, caused by house dust mite.

Severe eye reactions

Allergic keratoconjunctivitis is a more serious allergic eye disease often occurring in the young and needing intensive therapy, as not only are the symptoms far more exaggerated but the condition is sight-threatening and prompt effective treatment is imperative to reduce the risk of poor vision and blindness.[10]

Nose

The nose is the main mode by which we breathe in air and the allergens it contains. One of the main functions of the nose is to filter inspired air, so that most of the allergens we inhale stay within the nose – hence nose allergy is a very common problem. Allergy in the nose causes the condition known as rhinitis, an inflammation of the mucous membranes which is characterised by three symptoms: blockage, runny nose and sneezing.

Hay fever

Seasonal allergic rhinitis is more commonly known as hay fever – up to 40 per cent of us have had this condition, which is also associated with sleep disturbance and resultant excessive daytime sleepiness. The condition is so prevalent that car insurance companies are beginning to penalise sufferers as it is thought that over two million drivers have accidents, near misses or experience loss of control of the vehicle as a direct result of hay fever.[11] Research conducted by Halfords showed that at least 27 per cent of British motorists suffer from streaming and swollen eyes, a runny nose and repeated sneezing. Alarming when we consider the number of bus, taxi, train and lorry operators, not to mention pilots, who will suffer in exactly the same way.

Many patients who suffer from rhinitis symptoms, in particular excessive mucus (rhinorrhoea; post-nasal drip), feel that giving up milk products makes them better. This is despite negative allergy testing and the fact that food allergy very rarely affects the nose. It is due to a perception that milk and nose mucus have similar qualities and that ingesting the former leads to the latter. It is the same with sinus symptoms, which patients typically describe as blockage, or a full feeling in the face. Yet there is no relation to dairy product allergy. A runny or blocked nose after eating foods such as cheese or drinking red wine is much more likely due to histamine present in the food than allergy. Furthermore, nose tingling and running after eating horseradish, mustard or chilli peppers is due to molecules in the aroma of the foods irritating the lining of the nose directly, causing a rejection reaction rather like allergy but by direct stimulation of receptors instead.

There is vastly less mystery around inhaled allergies when we compare them to the endless nuances of food allergy which we will discuss. And the advice to combat them follows suit. Avoidance is key but unfortunately it can be problematic, as it involves really understanding the nature of the allergens that affect you – rather than simply avoiding certain foodstuffs.

Now that you have a good understanding of inhaled allergies, in the workouts below we give a full run-through of avoidance strategies; available medical treatments but also some failsafe measures you can employ in your own home to minimise and remedy outbreaks.

Diagnose, Avoid and Remedy

Notice

If you have jumped straight to this section, then welcome! The mentality for a quick and easy fix is something we have anticipated, which is why the routines below are not only short but useable without reading any other element of this guide. However, achieving maximum results can only come from a sufficient awareness of the nuances involved with inhaled allergies. Therefore, please take a few minutes to flick back to the outline above.

Diagnosis

- Blood test
- Skin prick test

- ### *Blood test*

Your GP will have some samples drawn from your blood. The test is looking at mixes of specific IgE antibodies – as discussed above, these are the antibodies relating to, and causing, allergy. Groups of common allergens such as tree pollens, grass pollens, animal dander, house dust mite and moulds are tested together. If a group shows significant levels of antibody, implying allergy, a second test on that particular mix is performed looking at each individual antigen, e.g. different types of grass pollen from the grass mix group, to see which actual grass type the patient reacts to. This process is carried out for all of the mixes. A total IgE (the total number of antibodies in the blood) can be asked for – if it is very high, but all of the mixes are negative, it means the doctor has to look further for the antigen (allergen), or consider parasitic infection – another cause of a very high total IgE level, along with multiple myeloma – a rare blood cancer. It is worth noting that a number of factors can impact the results of the test – in particular smoking. Make sure prior to the test your GP is aware that you smoke or if you have spent a long period of time in any countries where parasitic infections are relatively common.

- ### *Skin prick test*

Once the results of the blood tests come through, additional testing with skin prick is recommended for those antigens that have appeared as positive on the blood test. This is to examine the severity of the reaction – how the patient actually responds to the allergen may not be predicted by the level of the IgE antibody. Plus rarer types of allergy not included in the mixes can easily be tested with skin prick, particularly if there is no specific IgE antibody test (there are hundreds, but there are many millions of things you could be allergic to). Skin prick or skin scratch tests are a very common method of understanding inhaled allergens. They are also very cheap and straightforward to perform and the results are immediate. The basic premise is that these tests contain extracts of house dust mite, cat, dog, mould spores, grass and tree pollen. When inoculated into the skin you are looking for a 'weal' or 'flare',[12] which is a sign of an inflammatory response – allergy. This weal is then compared to a positive control, which is when histamine is also directly inoculated into the skin...

Avoid

- *Simple but effective avoidance of triggers*

The key to avoidance is knowing what to avoid, so the tests above are very important. Tree and grass pollen, along with that of other plants such as weeds, are hard to avoid. Remember, pollen counts are at their highest in early morning and early evening – so keep the windows closed at those times. Moulds are particularly present in autumn with rotting leaves and foliage, but also commonly appear in old houses with slightly rotting timbers, which are made worse if damp conditions prevail. House dust mite is by far the most common allergen – the allergy is actually to proteins found in dust mite faeces. Home environments that are warm and windy are ideal, since you can keep the windows open during the day, stopping a build-up of dust. Concentrate on the bedroom. Avoid carpets and always dust with a damp cloth so the dust is absorbed. Avoid feather duvets and pillows; have a sealed dust cover over your mattress. Sealed stone floors or tiled floors are preferable – certainly no rugs. Use a particulate filter system (e.g. a HEPA filter) and have a dust filter fitted to your vacuum cleaner.

A more extreme way of avoiding these items is to move location – perhaps to somewhere mountainous, dry and arid.

Avoidance is just as much about vigilance in the moment and steering clear of triggers as it is about taking steps each and every day to mitigate the severity of outbreaks. All too often we see allergy and intolerance cause symptoms far more severe than necessary because the body is just not kept in good working order – in particular due to lack of good sleep, optimal hydration and a balanced diet. While the defences of a sufferer are naturally lower, the techniques below will begin the process of immune system repair – which means that your body has a chance to rejuvenate naturally, so put yourself in the best situation to begin with.

Wash your hair and body before you go to bed

Most people take a shower when they wake up in the morning. This is an understandable routine but it is essential in relation to inhaled allergies that you shower just before you go to bed – especially in the build-up to and through the allergy season. Sufferers often complain of waking up feeling puffy, blocked and generally not in great spirits. The reason for this is that the pollen and host of other inhaled triggers get trapped in the hair and on the body during the day. Without washing this out you essentially incubate yourself for eight to ten hours a night in the very thing you are trying to avoid. This, of course, also applies to anyone you share your bed with. Focus on regular cleaning of bed clothes and bed linen – this will get rid of dust, pollen and spores which may accumulate.

Act before you react

As we will discuss shortly, there are numerous drugs and sprays that effectively remedy the symptoms of inhaled allergy. In terms of avoidance, the point here is to adopt a routine of acting before you react: this means that if you know you are susceptible to certain seasons or animals, it is essential that you proactively take your medicines – don't wait to react when it's too late to avoid an outbreak. So the time to get your body primed with antihistamine or a depot injection of steroid (see page 37) is in the weeks leading up to the hay fever season for example – and not at the first signs of watering eyes and a runny nose.

In consultation with your GP, map out exactly when you suffer throughout the year. This means you are crystal clear about the 'act' phase, but the consultation might also make you aware of certain irritants you weren't conscious of at other points in the year.

You might find it useful to note down your personal experience of when seasonal allergy strikes as it will vary slightly for different people across the country. Take a standard calendar and note down:

- When early signs start (runny nose, congestion or itching eyes)
- The time of day that causes the most discomfort
- Duration of your season
- The point where symptoms subside

On your next consultation with your GP take this valuable information along and together you can work out exactly when your 'act' phase must begin.

Honey does not work! (At least not in the way they say)

There has been a long-standing argument which says a teaspoon of honey a day will prevent allergic responses to pollen, as the honey itself contains pollens you react to and early exposure helps dampen down the response. As sweet as the advice is it is unfortunately not true, as grass and tree pollens aren't sources of nectar, which is what the bees are really after. There is almost no pollen in nectar, which is what honey is made of. However, those who swear by honey as an effective remedy simply have their cause and effect wrong. Honey is a powerful immune booster and one teaspoon a day will have a positive effect on rebalancing your body's natural defences. Honey in small doses has also long been promoted as a tool to encourage the body into restful sleep – which combined with the sleep hygiene routine above ensures the maximum rest and repair the body needs.

Don't cut nasal hairs and eyebrows too short

Trimming bushy eyebrows and protruding nasal hairs is a very normal cosmetic activity. But remember these outcrops of hair serve a very important function in preventing airborne allergens from entering the body. The hairs above the eye stop particles from entering the conjunctiva and hypersensitive nasal hairs act both as a defensive wall and a signal to sneeze and expel anything they come into contact with.

Trimming both areas is still okay, so don't panic. The point is to trim only a few millimetres and under no circumstances wax or remove all hair completely, as you then leave your body's most vulnerable areas completely unprotected.

Remedy

Medical therapy is in theory pretty straightforward in the sense that the inflammatory response needs to be blocked, so that the effects of histamine and the other inflammatory mediators produced are negated. What is less straightforward is a clear regime that indicates when to use which treatment or combination of treatments.

- **Take control**

The best way to plan a remedy regime is by following what is known as the 'Ladder of intervention'. Different people will respond differently to each stage of the ladder, some not needing to advance beyond steps 1 or 2. On the other hand, some might get the best respite from the latter stages. Either way, it is important to start at the first step and then move down.

Ladder of intervention – nose allergy, whether seasonal (hay fever) or perennial

1. Salt water douche
2. Salves on the nose e.g. Vaseline
3. Steroid/antihistamine sprays and eye drops
4. Mast cell stabilising sprays and eye drops
5. Antihistamine tablet
6. Antileucotriene tablet
7. Course of high dose steroid tablets
8. Depot injection of steroids

Salt water douche or washout   Salt water washouts for the nose are not to be underestimated as these agents help to remove the dust, pollen and debris we collect during the day and night, to which we are actively allergic. For nose allergy (hay fever/rhinitis), you can regularly wash the nose out, getting rid of all these particles which stick inside the nose as part of its filtration function. For this, use salt water. Take half a teaspoon of table salt and dissolve it in one cup of boiled tap water. Let it cool to room temperature. Then, using the palm of your hand as a bowl, close one of your nostrils with your finger, just pushing on the outside, then bring your open nostril to your palm and sniff up some salt water, blowing it out after a few seconds. Repeat for both sides. This is the basic exercise. However, even better is to use a 5ml syringe without a needle (your pharmacy will have these) and draw up 5ml of salt water, then gently spray it into the nose in four different positions:

1.   Lying on your back

2.   Lying on your left side

3.   Lying on your right side

4.   Lying face down on a table, head over one end, peering at the underside of the table (we know this one is a bit hard!)

On all occasions, let the salt water wash into your nose, and blow it out after a few seconds. This is particularly good for house dust mite allergy, which is the most common allergy you can have – it's best done twice a day, before going to bed and when waking up. Even if symptoms subside we recommend continuing this process daily as a preventative measure.

Nasal salves   Very simply adding a salve or petroleum jelly such as Vaseline to the entrance and interior of the nose will minimise the harmful particles that are able to enter the nasal passage and provoke a reaction. This is essential in providing protection throughout the night, but it works fantastically in conjunction with other daytime remedies such as the salt water douche or the nasal spray regime.

Sprays and eye drops   Antihistamine is available as a nose spray for nose allergy, as eye drops for eye allergy or as tablets for lung/skin/gut allergy. It can also be used intravenously for more severe cases of allergy. Sodium cromoglycate is also available as a spray, as drops and in inhaler form. It is used for allergy in the nose, eyes or lungs. It stabilises mast cells, stopping them releasing histamine, and therefore prevents the symptoms of an itch or a runny nose, for example. Steroid nose sprays are also very useful, as steroids dampen down the inflammatory pathway in an highly effective, but poorly understood way. In bad cases of nose allergy, a combination spray of antihistamine and steroid together can be very effective (there is no combination spray with sodium cromoglycate as well).

Antihistamine tablets   Antihistamines typically come in two forms, Drowsy and Non-drowsy, but the labelling is not always clear. Drowsy medicines will make you feel tired and sleepy so are not ideal for daytime use – but they are often recommended for night-time use to promote restful sleep. Your GP will be able to make sure you have the most suitable medication but the active ingredients are as follows:

* *Drowsy*: Chlorphenamine, Hydroxyzine and Promethazine
* *Non-Drowsy*: Cetirizine, Loratadine and Fexofenadine

Antileucotrienes   Initially devised as anti-asthma drugs, these agents can be very helpful in blocking the leucotriene effect of allergy. Usually in conjunction with steroid and antihistamine sprays, they are designed for long-term usage.

Course of high dose steroid tablets   Steroids are the most widely used drugs to combat allergy. They affect metabolism and the distribution of T and B lymphocytes. The idea is that the medication mimics the effect of the stress hormone cortisol, which is excreted from the adrenal gland to minimise the effects of inflammation in the body. They are very effective in the treatment of allergy, whichever part of the body it affects.

Systemic (tablet form) steroids are intended primarily for short-term use only. Any course prescribed must be closely monitored by a trained professional and if you experience any side effects such as mania, vision changes, joint pain, anxiety or loss of appetite then contact them immediately. Don't worry, these symptoms are only temporary and often subside on their own, but keeping your GP in the loop means they can make small changes to dosage and drug type.

Depot injection of steroid   Depot injections are slow release, and circumvent, to a degree, the problem with giving higher doses of steroid tablets by mouth. Doses of 80–120mg are injected deep into the buttock muscle. This is released over 60–90 days, giving a daily dose of between 1 and 2 mg/day, as compared with a daily dose when giving high doses by mouth (above) of 40–50 mg/day. The alternative, of course, is to give a low maintenance dose of 1.5mg/day, by mouth.

The drugs you are prescribed are designed to last you the entire season and you are unlikely to build up a tolerance. If you do feel symptoms worsening even though you continue to adhere to your regime then consult with your GP, as there might be a change in the natural course of the condition and they can amend the medication accordingly.

Immunotherapy

This is a controversial topic and should only be considered in consultation with your GP. In immunotherapy treatment, a very small amount of the substance you are allergic to is given to you every day, rather like homeopathy. There is good evidence that this works for hay fever, but it is an arduous course to complete daily over three years and once the patient stops, symptoms that were reduced significantly start to reappear. It is also expensive: in the UK a three-year course costs around £9,000. The antigen (e.g. grass pollen in hay fever) can be given either under the tongue on special tiny pieces of sponge impregnated with the antigen or injected into the skin. The actual mode of action, like homeopathy, is not properly understood.

Immunotherapy is not a licensed treatment in the UK, but it is obvious that those with anaphylactic reactions to substances such as wasp stings, peanuts, etc., would greatly benefit from any reduction in the severity of their reaction. These anaphylaxis-inducing substances do not have an immunotherapy treatment yet, but much work is being done to try to develop one.

A Note on Asthma

Allergy is part of asthma. But it is so complex, multifactorial and potentially dangerous that it is beyond the scope of this book. However, if you do have an allergic component to your asthma then a basic understanding of diagnosis, avoidance and treatment is vital, but all remedy must be in consultation with your GP.

In Summary

Inhaled allergy sufferers are at risk from airborne agents which target the upper airways and the eyes. The outcome is seasonal or year-long physical and mental discomfort. Tackling it properly is a combination of pharmaceutical therapies (in consultation with your GP) and a strict regime of home remedy and avoidance.

4.

Ingested Allergies

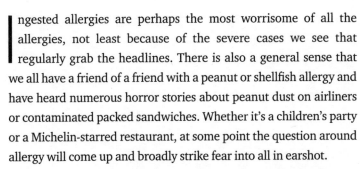

I ngested allergies are perhaps the most worrisome of all the allergies, not least because of the severe cases we see that regularly grab the headlines. There is also a general sense that we all have a friend of a friend with a peanut or shellfish allergy and have heard numerous horror stories about peanut dust on airliners or contaminated packed sandwiches. Whether it's a children's party or a Michelin-starred restaurant, at some point the question around allergy will come up and broadly strike fear into all in earshot.

You are no doubt reading this section because the dangers are at the forefront of your mind. If you or a family member actually do have a food allergy then stress levels are not only heightened but general advice is inconsistent, exacerbating the situation. This mindset is driven by a general assumption that in most cases food allergy results in death if not properly managed. The constant theme of this book is that in reality, this anxiety is because of a fear of the unknown and is not necessarily representative of any statistical danger to you or your family. That is not to say that extreme cases don't happen. They do. But so infrequent are they that it really is quite amazing how convincingly they drive the overall story.

The chapter that follows is designed to outline the real dangers of allergy as distinct from intolerance and provide clear-cut and simple advice on how to avoid, prevent and remedy ingested allergies, giving you back control and true peace of mind.

What is a Food Allergy?

Food allergy is when your immune system reacts to foods, which then causes inflammation of the body's tissues. Actual food allergy is rare and tends to run in the family. An estimated 5 per cent of adults have a food allergy, compared with about 8 per cent of children. And while some children outgrow allergies – usually those to milk, eggs and wheat – many retain their allergies through adulthood.[13]

Once you have become sensitised to a food, just like with pollen or any other allergen, you react every time you eat that food, as the antibodies that bind to the food you are allergic to lie in wait and then bind to mast cells in the mucosa of the gut. Unfortunately, doctors are unable to predict the severity of any future reaction. This means symptoms that are mild on the first reaction can be serious the next time. It is therefore essential that any early signs of flare-ups, or indeed history of allergy in the family, are reported to a medical practitioner.

Common Food Allergens

The most common foods that prompt an allergic response are the proteins found in:

- Cow's milk
- Eggs
- Tree nuts
- Wheat
- Soy
- Fish
- Shellfish
- Peanuts

Usually we are allergic to only a tiny fraction of the available foodstuffs out there in the world. The effect of ingesting something genuinely hazardous (such as a toxin) is something the body is constantly on guard against and extremely sensitive to – food allergy in particular comes from us being almost oversensitive, so we default to reacting too much rather than too little.

Unfortunately, food allergy is a vastly over-diagnosed condition – not only because of the confusion with food intolerance but also because of the great trend for introspection and self-diagnosis (Doctor Google). Classically, if a patient is allergic to a foodstuff, they will develop tingling and itchiness in the mouth and throat immediately after eating it. When the added effect of underlying allergy is present, for example that of grass pollen, the mouth and lips may swell, and extreme itchiness can occur. This is called the iceberg effect, because while these symptoms are the visible tip the underlying allergy is hidden beneath the surface. In fact, the patient is allergic to birch pollen and has hay fever, but nuts like hazelnuts (found in a lot of other foodstuffs) mimic the pollen structure of birch, and so cause mouth symptoms when eating. This is not life-threatening, but can cause real panic, because the symptoms can be misdiagnosed, or simply mistaken by the patient, as anaphylaxis. It is otherwise known as Oral Allergy Syndrome – see below.

For the GP or attending doctor, the patient's or their parents' history of reaction to food will often be exaggerated, wrongly described and/or self-diagnosed. This can be to the extent that the doctor cannot categorically say that the patient, although possibly allergic, did or did not suffer an anaphylactic reaction, because the consequences of true anaphylaxis, though incredibly rare (such as death from peanut ingestion), are so severe. So often the doctor must go along with the patient's/parents' diagnosis, and it is written into their medical notes, often becoming fact before any tests have been done to confirm or deny even allergy, let alone anaphylaxis.

This might sound a little scathing, but the point is your health is the focus here. Tempting as it may be, try to keep an open mind and remember, by staving off putting yourself through the mental anguish of self-diagnosis, you will bring about quicker and more effective solutions to medical issues.

If you or a family member are experiencing reactions to certain foods – or indeed to any category discussed in this book – then first of all please read on, as it will help ease your mind. But also make a note of all things that cause symptoms, or those substances you are just worried about consuming for fear of symptoms, and take this to your GP. Try to remember all the other things you've eaten in conjunction with the item you are concerned about. This gives the medical professional great data to work with and they can then act quickly and organise the most accurate and appropriate testing.

Oral Allergy Syndrome

Unfortunately, the exaggerated border control required to protect us from truly bad things means that proteins similar to – but not the same as – those that trigger an allergic response can themselves trick the body and still cause an allergic reaction. For example, if you are allergic to ragweed (a flowering shrub common across subtropical and tropical parts of the world) then you may also develop reactions to bananas or melons.[14] This is known as cross-reactivity. Cross-reactivity for other allergens is not common but when foods specifically are the cause of the immune confusion we call this 'oral allergy syndrome (OAS)'.[15] Classically it occurs when patients already suffering from hay fever caused by allergy to birch tree pollen then eat a foodstuff they are allergic to, or one that mimics one of the birch pollen core antigens. Classically this is hazelnut protein, which mimics the Bet vi core antigen in birch pollen. This is another instance of the iceberg effect – the symptoms may only be felt in the mouth due to ingestion of nut protein, but there is a great degree of underlying antibody from the birch pollen hay fever. Outside the hay fever season, no symptoms may be felt when eating any of the food allergens listed below.

With this in mind get into the habit of noting down any time when your seasonal symptoms are much worse than usual – or if you experience any unusual tingling in the mouth. In particular, consider if your symptoms worsen in relation to eating any of the following foods:

- **Birch pollen:** apple, almond, carrot, celery, cherry, hazelnut, kiwi, peach, pear, plum
- **Grass pollen:** celery, melons, oranges, peaches, tomato

If you notice a trend or even if you are a huge tomato fan and are now a bit worried, again note down exactly the foods which seem to be causing an increase in seasonal symptoms – or a tingling sensation in the mouth – and then book an appointment with your GP.

Food Intolerance

We are going to set in stone a controversial marker. Food intolerance is not allergy. Why the need for this seemingly unnecessary distinction? A Google search for 'food intolerance' produces a huge range of opinions and advice, which make it appear a very difficult and complex subject. This is unhelpful, as in fact food intolerance is something that can be identified, managed and avoided with some very simple, clear routines based on a real understanding of the problem. It is our mission to stop the terms 'allergy' and 'intolerance' from becoming interchangeable or synonymous.

So, once again: intolerance is not allergy. Food intolerance is an abnormal reaction when consuming foods which pose no threat to the body, and whilst the symptoms sound similar to allergy, they are limited to:

- Bloating
- Migraines
- Headaches
- Coughing
- Runny nose
- Feeling under the weather
- Stomach ache
- Irritable bowel – cramping pains and diarrhoea

A far more useful way of describing intolerance would be simply to say one has difficulty in digesting certain foodstuffs (and/or the chemicals and proteins within them). There is no attempt here to downplay the impact of food intolerance – indeed, some cases can exhibit symptoms verging on those seen in allergy. But while unpleasant, rest assured that they are unlikely to result in death or even come close, and therefore it is essential to adopt the mindset *reduce the stress, reduce the symptoms*. A good distinction here is that an allergic reaction is an immediate medical problem, while an intolerance affects the body over a long period of time, though can cause serious damage to, say, the intestines if not treated correctly.

The brain does not hesitate to play tricks on itself, so a true understanding of the dangers or lack thereof is a huge step towards calmly resolving the issue – rather than pacing around the room preparing to take a scalpel to your own throat when you have only over-peppered the chicken and chorizo soup. The plan here is to get out of the immediate danger mindset and think calmly, safe in the knowledge that you know the measures you can take to minimise and even prevent the effect intolerances can have in the long term.

Lactose Intolerance and Lactase Insufficiency

Arnold Schwarzenegger famously said: 'Milk is for babies. When you grow up you have to drink beer.' Babies don't have teeth for their first year, so all their nutrients have to come in liquid form. Milk is a very good way of achieving this. While the advice is a little crude, the sentiment raises a very important point – a baby's ability to digest milk. Infants produce high levels of lactase in the stomach. This is the enzyme that allows the body to digest lactose – the sugars found in milk and milk products.

During early development, of course, the staple for babies is breast milk – but as they are weaned off the breast their available lactase is still enough to sufficiently break down and digest cow's milk and receive the benefit of the nutrients and growth hormones it contains. But overall, about 75 per cent of the world's population lose some of their lactase enzymes after weaning.[16] And in some cases, where people can become lactose intolerant, lactase production drops further, and although the growing child moves on to solid food there may come a point where the stomach can no longer sufficiently break down these sugars. This is intolerance defined – the inability to digest certain foods. Broadly, we are all lactose intolerant to varying degrees, for reasons outlined above. Generally, lactose intolerance will manifest itself as discomfort and pain after eating milk-derived products, as well as bloating and diarrhoea.

Milk-derived products

- **The obvious**
  Milk
  Cheese
  Ice cream
  Butter
  Yoghurt
  Cream

- **The less obvious**
  Chocolate
  Biscuits
  Salad creams, dressings and mayonnaise
  Boiled sweets

Cake
Some breads and baked goods
Breakfast cereals
Instant-mix potatoes and soup
Some processed or canned meats
Pancakes, muffins, etc., made with sachet mix

If the symptoms described above sound familiar then it is important to root out precisely which item or combination of items you are intolerant to. The most effective way of exploring this is to stop all dairy completely and see if the symptoms subside. Remember that a number of foods might contain dairy or trace amounts of it without you being aware. To really get to the bottom of the problem if symptoms persist, follow the advice below about exclusion dieting. Major changes to your diet will have positive effects but best to inform your GP prior to embarking on such a regime.

Gluten Intolerance and Coeliac Disease

It is commonplace to hear the phrase: 'I am allergic to gluten.' Hopefully, by this stage you are coming to the realisation that this statement is almost certainly misguided, given the rarity of such a condition. Granted, if the person genuinely does have an allergy related to gluten then make sure you hide the bagels immediately. The point here is to once again reaffirm that often (indeed, 98 per cent of the time) your comrade will be describing and suffering from a gluten intolerance, or coeliac disease. These terms are very nearly synonymous – so close, in fact, that any gluten intolerance that falls outside the remit of coeliac disease is defined as non-coeliac gluten sensitivity (NCGS). The key departure is that while NCGS can result in the same symptoms, with the same severity as coeliac disease, the immune response that causes them is different. In fact, NCGS appears to be nothing to do with the immune system as there are no associated antibodies or damage to the lining of the gut.

Coeliac disease involves products of gluten digestion (gliadin) linking with genetically programmed T lymphocytes – a type of white blood cell that plays a key role in the body's immune system. These T lymphocytes live in the wall of the gut. This linking process produces inflammatory hormones (cytokines), which lead to changes in the bowel lining and the symptoms of coeliac disease. This is a type 4 hypersensitivity reaction, whereas allergy, for example hay fever, is a type 1 hypersensitivity reaction – so they are similar, but not the same. Part of this process involves deficiency in the enzyme tissue transglutaminase (tTG), which is there to help reduce inflammation and ease swelling. In the case of coeliac disease, however, this enzyme further breaks down the gliadin, which in turn further promotes the T cells to produce even more inflammatory hormones, rather than reducing them: a vicious cycle.

This is all made worse by the immunity part of the disease. Remember, immunity is the body's natural process of being exposed to microdoses of harmful outside influences, so that it can protect itself and become immune on its next encounter. Here, however, the patient instead creates an antibody to tTG, which binds with tTG in the gut wall. The creation of antibodies to your own body cells is called autoimmunity and is a type 5 hypersensitivity reaction, allergy being a type 1 hypersensitivity. So coeliac disease is a combination of types 4 and 5 hypersensitivity, but again, is not allergy.

This antibody to tTG – known as anti-tTG – can be measured in the blood, and is therefore a good diagnostic sign for coeliac disease.

From here on in we will describe only coeliac disease, but the distinction is important to make if only to remind ourselves that symptoms can be indicative of almost anything – but the implications can be vast – so take the right actions as guided by this book, to understand your reactions.

Getting tested

With an incidence of up to one in two hundred people, coeliac disease is a common form of food intolerance and describes inflammation of the small intestine, resulting in the inability to absorb and make use of nutrients. More specifically, it is a disease where affected individuals have a genetic predisposition to react to gliadin – a protein that is part of gluten. Tests for this include biopsy of the gut lining and blood tests that look at the HLA class of genes, or antibodies to transglutaminase – the enzyme responsible.

There is no way around it. An intestinal biopsy is not fun. It is relatively painless but it does involve taking some samples of the small intestinal lining. A scope is inserted through the mouth and down the oesophagus, stomach and into the small intestine. This is certainly invasive but the good news is that this is very much an outpatient, or same-day, procedure, so there will be no stay in hospital needed.

Screenings of this kind will be conducted by a specialist physician, who will also request annual check-ups to monitor progress and highlight any nutritional abnormalities.

If you think that you might have coeliac disease or feel any of the reactions or discomforts mentioned thus far, visit your GP.

Histamine Intolerance

Histamine causes swelling or dilation in the blood vessels to help target white blood cells directly towards a point of external attack, since as a blood vessel widens flow increases, as does vessel wall permeability, causing leakage of fluid into tissue – swelling. This blocks off outward draining (into the body) lymphatic fluid temporarily, due to local pressure effects. Imagine being stung on the lip by a bee. You see a reaction as your lip doubles, even quadruples, in size. This is the body sectioning off the attack – and in effect saying 'nothing to see here' as it quarantines the problem and the remaining bodily function goes about its normal business. Putting two and two together, it is clear what the pharmaceutical remedy to excessive histamine release is. You guessed it: an antihistamine.

Histamine intolerance, then, describes the point at which the body is in histamine overload – or has too much of it. The implications of histamine intolerance, such as from eating food containing histamine, are very serious because histamine enters the bloodstream quickly – and the effect can therefore reach nearly every extremity of the human body. Once again, the underlying issue here is that some patients are unable to sufficiently break down ingested (eaten) histamine, leaving some residual surplus that causes a delta of symptoms, from nausea and vomiting to hives and easy sexual arousal. Yes, you read this correctly. Histamines have a vasodilation effect (a widening of the blood vessels). This has the immediate effect of a higher libido – and the side effect of more easily achieving an orgasm. But before you start praying for histamine intolerance the reality is that an unprompted raising of your sexual interest is a major cause for anxiety, and in men is a cause of premature ejaculation. Sexual dysfunctions can be incredibly difficult personally and for couples and partners. The pressure some individuals feel can be overwhelming and it can often leave someone feeling helpless as it seems so out of their control. The good news is that this might be evidence of high levels of histamine circulating in the blood – in which case an exclusion diet will once again uncover this and then resolve the issue entirely.

Histamine-rich foods

It might surprise you that while we generally think of histamine as a chemical generated by the body, there are in fact several histamine-rich foods which, in those unable to sufficiently break the chemical down, add to the problem of surplus. Foodstuffs such as fish as it begins to decompose (often the cause of self-diagnosed fish allergy) and fermented alcoholic beverages, especially red wines, champagnes and cask ales, are major culprits. The latter in particular can cause anything from mild reactions to severe abdominal pain. These are relatively well known, but there exists an alarmingly long yet essential list of far more offensive items which histamine-intolerant people must be made aware of:

- **Fermented foods**
  Sauerkraut
  Vinegar (and vinegar-containing foods)
  Soy sauce
  Kefir (fermented milk)
  Yoghurt
  Kombucha teas
  Kimchi

- **Cured meats**
  Bacon
  Salami
  Pepperoni
  Luncheon meats
  Hotdogs

- **Soured foods**
  Sour cream
  Sour milk
  Buttermilk
  Sourdough

- **Dried fruits and cheeses**
  Apricots
  Prunes
  Dates
  Figs
  Raisins
  Most citrus fruits
  Any aged cheese; goat's
  cheese

- **Nuts and vegetables**
  Walnuts
  Peanuts
  Cashews
  Avocados
  Aubergines (eggplants)
  Spinach
  Tomatoes

- **Fish**
  All smoked fish
  Mackerel
  Mahi-mahi
  Tuna
  Anchovies
  Sardines

This makes grim reading for any sufferer who enjoys … well, basically anything worth enjoying – but those affected are in the minority. Studies of incidence range from 1–8 per cent[17] in terms of population prevalence – highlighting our near infancy in truly understanding histamine intolerance.

These listed items may cause a marked anaphylaxis-type response in histamine-susceptible people – note once again that this is *not* allergy, although patients often describe it as such and refuse to believe it is not allergy as the symptoms include flushing, palpitations and urticarial rash (a type of skin rash with raised itchy bumps).

This histamine sensitivity comes from a deficiency of the enzyme diamine oxidase, which breaks down histamine. Lack of this enzyme is said to occur in 1 per cent of the population, with 80 per cent of sufferers said to be middle-aged. *Diagnosis can only be achieved by an exclusion diet*, although a blood test for diamine oxidase levels can be performed The full breakdown of the step-by-step exclusion protocol is laid out below.

Toxins and Chemicals in Food

Finally, we must briefly outline the last realm of intolerance, which comprises those foods containing certain toxins and chemicals that, once again, elicit a bodily response. The obvious starting point is foods exposed to pesticides during cultivation – and this is why it is essential to thoroughly wash fruit and salad items before consuming them. The same is true of naturally occurring toxins such as aflatoxin, which is found in legumes and beans. Again, a thorough soaking prior to cooking should reduce the harmful levels almost entirely, but you must be vigilant.

The most important chemicals to understand are amines. These are biologically active molecules and are derivatives of ammonia. The most notable amine is tyramine, which is a similar compound to histamine and therefore causes the same subset of symptoms and concerns when ingested in those lacking diamine oxidase, the enzyme responsible for breaking down histamine.

Foods containing considerable amounts of tyramine include meats that are potentially spoiled or pickled; some fish, poultry and beef that has been aged, smoked, fermented or marinated;

and most pork (except cured ham). Other foods include chocolate, alcoholic beverages and fermented foods, processed meat, most cheeses (except ricotta, cottage, cream and soft cheese with a rind), sour cream, yoghurt, shrimp paste, soy sauce, soybean condiments, teriyaki sauce, tempeh, miso soup, sauerkraut, kimchi, broad (fava) beans, green bean pods, Italian flat (Romano) beans, snow peas, edamame, avocados, bananas, pineapples, aubergines, figs, red plums, raspberries, peanuts, Brazil nuts, coconuts, yeast and an array of cacti and other plants.

Some people are more sensitive to these than others and an allergic-type reaction can ensue. Of particular importance is that the chemical make-up of tyramine (a monoamine) means that patients can have an extreme reaction to tyramine-containing foods when they are taking a prescribed drug containing monoamine oxidase inhibitors (MAOIs), such as in a patient taking the antidepressant drug Moclobemide, for example. This inhibits monoamine oxidase, an enzyme in the brain that breaks down monoamines, which are also involved in nerve function. It is important to avoid tyramine- and histamine-containing food if on this form of medication, otherwise very high levels can occur in the brain – with potentially serious consequences.

Other foods with chemicals causing direct irritant effects are horseradish, mustard and chilli peppers. This is due to molecules in the aroma of the foods irritating the lining of the nose directly, causing a rejection reaction in terms of mucus production – rather like allergy, but by direct stimulation of the receptors instead. In chilli, this chemical is capsaicin; in mustard and horseradish it is allyl isothiocyanate. Nose-watering and sometimes sneezing with certain foods such as these may also be due to a reflex initiated by receptors in the mouth.

Salicylates, sulphates and additives are perhaps the best-known chemicals, as they are present in numerous foods, especially processed and preserved foods. This being the case, they are also likely to be the hardest to avoid. So be sure to understand the contents of salicylic acid-containing foods, especially if you are asthmatic or intolerant to aspirin.

Processed meats and foods high in MSG (monosodium glutamate) and other flavour enhancers contain other additives that can cause a bodily reaction to eating them.

And finally, a German study found that 7 per cent of people had an intolerance to wine: red, white or rosé. This is not because of the grapes, but rather due to the sulphites and colourings used in the ageing process – they found the largest reactions were to carmine (red) and annatto (yellow).

As you can see, the amount of information available on allergy and intolerance is staggering, and as we dig a little deeper into the concepts we are engulfed by complex medical terminology. The purpose thus far has been to highlight that while on the surface this seems inaccessible and complicated, offering you some ways to understand the chemistry here makes for much easier reading. Importantly, in the pages that follow we show you how this knowledge can be put into step-by-step prevention measures and effective remedies.

In getting to this stage it should now be clear that there is a stark and important difference between allergy and intolerance – and your mind should also be eased that you, your loved ones and your friends are very likely to be sufferers of the latter.

The Microbiome

The whole discussion of food allergy and intolerance would be entirely inadequate without awareness of one very important factor, one you wouldn't normally think of – the huge mass of bacteria within the gut, which forms its own mini ecosystem: the microbiome. This mass of bacteria, parasites, viruses and other bugs lives in a functional syncytium (win–win relationship) with the human body, carrying out many symbiotic vital functions. Its presence is the reason why the gut contains 80 per cent of the lymphatic tissue of the body, as it has to be constantly fighting off toxins and organisms trying to enter the body through the gut lining – which in an adult male covers an area the size of two doubles tennis courts.

The gut microbiome is estimated to consist of over twenty trillion organisms and weighs in at around 2kg. It is for this reason that any exclusion diet or dietary analysis is flawed, albeit possibly to a minor degree, as these organisms take ingested food and partially digest it into other compounds – the effects of which are very hard to determine as they are so varied.

Diagnose, Avoid and Remedy

Diagnosing food allergy

- Skin prick testing
- Blood testing
- Tests to avoid

• *Skin prick testing*

The good thing about food allergy is that the antibodies that bind to certain foods, causing the allergic response, are present all over the body, in the mast cell areas already discussed: nose, throat, eye lining, gut, skin, lungs – the surfaces that are exposed to the outside world. So skin prick testing for allergy is both relevant and easy. It is the best test. Positive and negative controls are needed to compare – the positive control is histamine, which *will* cause a reaction unless there is a major immune response problem; the negative control is water.

The food or substance that the patient considers they may be allergic to is pricked into the skin, ideally on the inside surface of the forearm. One of the best ways to do this is to bring the food in its purest form: a stick of celery, a kiwi fruit, a peanut, etc. The nurse or doctor will prick the food, then immediately prick it into the skin, in a pre-marked place, next to the positive and negative controls. After a period of ten minutes, the pricked areas are examined under a magnifying glass and the response noted. What we are looking for is the diameter of the swelling (weal). This is then compared to the positive control – the reaction caused by the histamine (usually around 5mm) – and the negative control – the reaction caused by the water (0mm). Many foodstuffs and other common allergens, like house dust mite, pollen, yeast, animal hair, etc., are also available in purified form in bottles from companies producing allergy-testing medical kits – but, still, the fresh product is best. Remember, if you are taking immunity-reducing drugs like antihistamines, antileukotrienes or steroids, this test will not work – you need to avoid taking them for a week, if possible.

• *Blood testing*

The other way of testing for allergy is a blood test looking for specific IgE antibodies to individual foods. There is a wide range of allergens (240 and counting) to which the gold standard immunoCAP process for testing has been applied. The antigen – i.e. an allergen such as peanut – is bound to a fluorescent molecule in a testing area. Blood from the patient is then applied to the testing area. If the blood contains antibodies to peanut the antibodies bind to the antigen and its molecule, which then changes both its shape and the colour of its fluorescence – so it can be identified. The more fluorescent this new colour the more antibodies exist in the blood and the greater the degree of allergy – in theory. Although this test appears to be quite scientific, and less subjective than skin prick testing, it is in fact inferior, as it depends on the quality of the testing areas produced by the company making the machine, which are known to be variable. The level of response will also vary depending on whether the patient has recently been exposed to the substance they are allergic to.

• *Tests to avoid*

An associated test, called total IgE, which measures the total level of IgE antibody in the blood, is not as helpful, as it is very nonspecific and may also be related to parasitic or other infections, or malignancy such as myeloma. Furthermore, its level will change according to whether the patient has been exposed to the allergen recently – so the body's normal range is very hard to be certain of.

The facts are that allergy is a potentially serious issue and under-emphasising the need for proper medical investigations would be wholly unethical – not to mention potentially fatal.

Diagnosing intolerance – exclusion diet

There is only one good way to diagnose food intolerance, and that is to undergo an exclusion diet. Food allergy can also be tested this way, although the blood tests and skin prick tests above are more useful.

An exclusion diet means withdrawing all food except boiled peeled potatoes such as King Edward or Maris Piper (with no salt, butter or any other condiment) for three days and drinking water only. This will give you carbohydrate, some fibre, minerals, vitamins and water – enough to keep you going. Gut transit time, or the amount of time it takes for food to travel from your mouth through your digestive tract, is around 6–8 hours. Seventy-two hours should be enough to remove most residual foodstuffs from your body, notwithstanding the biome – see above.

At this point you can begin to reintroduce foodstuffs you feel you may be sensitive to. Keep a diary from the start of the exclusion diet of all the possible symptoms you think you may have that are related to eating food you are intolerant to. Abdominal pain, diarrhoea, distension, etc., should all be captured. And it's essential that you record your relaxed abdominal girth at the same level four times a day, at the same time.

- **Measuring abdominal girth**

    Hold the end of a fabric tape measure against your navel and then pass it around your waist, coming back to the same point. Take a big breath out and this will give you an accurate resting girth reading. Often you will not realise just how bloated you are as you may have become quite used to the feeling, so it goes unnoticed. Throughout the exclusion process you will be amazed at the daily reduction in measurement.

Eat boiled or mashed potatoes at the following times for three days and record your abdominal girth in the spaces below.

Drink at least 1.5 litres of water (not sparkling). On Days 1 and 2 you may experience a greater need to go to the loo as, by proxy, you are also detoxing.

	DAY 1	DAY 2	DAY 3
9 a.m.			
1 p.m.			
7 p.m.			

After three days, introduce the foodstuff you think you are allergic to. Note down the response – any tingling, swelling or an upset stomach, for example? Keep measuring abdominal girth and keep reintroducing new foods on a day-by-day basis.

Avoid

Food allergy is a straightforward allergy in a way, since avoidance, with due care and attention, is relatively clear-cut. However, foods are common anaphylaxis-inducing allergens, so this needs to be taken seriously. It perhaps goes without saying that avoidance is all about understanding exactly what you suffer from and ensuring you don't come into contact with it. It is also about constantly assisting your body with the simple and effective actions below, which means that symptoms can be minimised and even stopped entirely.

- ### Don't be gluten-free – be free from gluten

  The 'free from' movement has never been more prolific, with everything from gluten-free breads to mayonnaise. On the face of things this is a great lifeline for sufferers who want to maintain a near normal diet. The reality is that gluten-free foods are heavily packaged, overly-processed and by and large nutritionally void. Yes, you will avoid gluten but at the cost of leaving your body unloved and without the essential nutrient-rich foods which help repair, growth and most importantly immunity. Intolerance is a signal that your body is not quite aligned properly. Invest in yourself and eat clean (natural and unprocessed) foods and you might just find you aren't intolerant at all. This is certainly a longer-term remedy but it is essential given the effect intolerance can have on the body. This is particularly relevant for those who have been tested for gluten or any other sensitivities and whose results are negative – but whose symptoms persist.

- ### Take a moment and breathe

  It's important to remember that stress and anxiety *about* food intolerance are a major factor in worsening the symptoms *of* food intolerance. Rapid and shallow breathing will be common even without the patient knowing they are doing it. The issue here is that one is only breathing with the top of the chest and not drawing air correctly into the diaphragm.[18] Hyperventilation in itself leads to a host of issues including bloating, gas, diarrhoea, stomach and chest pain, which mimic and exacerbate the symptoms of food intolerance – and put the body under considerable duress. A daily routine of breathing exercises will rebalance a patient's natural response to symptoms from intolerance but also reduce associated symptoms, as drawing deep, controlled breaths into the diaphragm will stimulate the part of the nervous system responsible for relaxation.[19]

Each night before bed spend three minutes on the following exercise:

- Sit down on the edge of your bed.

- Make sure not to slouch and sit up as straight as possible with your shoulders relaxed.

- Close your eyes.

- Breathe in a deep slow breath through your nose. Try breathing in for at least ten seconds – longer if you can (easier after some practice).

- Then slowly breathe out through the mouth in an equally controlled manner, this time for at least fifteen seconds, and repeat six times or for three minutes (whichever comes first).

Again, avoidance is about managing allergy and intolerances, not constantly firefighting them as and when they strike. This strategy when adopted daily will significantly reduce the hysteria and also hugely reduce the symptoms.

In Summary

Food allergy and intolerance have been too closely linked and clearly marking out the differences is essential for you to understand exactly how you manage, treat and remedy outbreaks. Avoidance is the most essential message in living with allergy or intolerance and following simple daily actions brings great benefits to your health and mental well-being.

5.

Contact Allergies

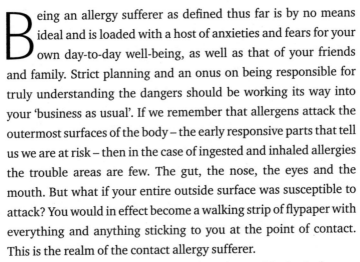

Being an allergy sufferer as defined thus far is by no means ideal and is loaded with a host of anxieties and fears for your own day-to-day well-being, as well as that of your friends and family. Strict planning and an onus on being responsible for truly understanding the dangers should be working its way into your 'business as usual'. If we remember that allergens attack the outermost surfaces of the body – the early responsive parts that tell us we are at risk – then in the case of ingested and inhaled allergies the trouble areas are few. The gut, the nose, the eyes and the mouth. But what if your entire outside surface was susceptible to attack? You would in effect become a walking strip of flypaper with everything and anything sticking to you at the point of contact. This is the realm of the contact allergy sufferer.

Allergy occurs predominantly on those parts of the body that are exposed to the outside world, primarily as a protective mechanism. Clearly the skin is very much one of those parts, so it has a profuse population of mast cells ready to bind to IgE and its antigen, whether a toxin or a microorganism. Broadly, contact allergy is part of the eczema spectrum of skin conditions. In reality, this is a catch-all term for a group of conditions that vary slightly in cause and effect but which all cause the skin to become red, itchy and inflamed. Usefully understanding, managing and preventing eczema means understanding the three most common manifestations:

1 Atopic (allergic) dermatitis (allergic contact)
2 Contact dermatitis
3 Irritant dermatitis

Atopic Dermatitis (Allergic Contact)

Firstly, some jargon busting. In the world of allergies, we often hear the term 'atopic'. Conditions such as atopic asthma or hay fever spring to mind but this also applies to some forms of dermatitis. 'Atopic' simply means the presence of 'atopy' – one's underlying allergy problem. Asthma, hay fever and dermatitis form what is known as the atopic triad,[20] as if you have a natural predisposition (or family history) towards one condition you are likely to be at risk of both other atopic disorders.

Someone with atopic dermatitis, then, was always destined to have the ailment beyond the age of five. Similar to our breakdown of lactose intolerance, we are all born with eczema as part of the body's natural immune maturation process. Branches of eczema are a mainstay of infant life with redness and rashes appearing primarily on the cheeks and scalp but often spreading to the legs and chest. After about the age of one, the symptoms are also likely to appear on the elbows, wrists and ankles.[21] As described above, this is the process of the body encountering a host of new particles and working out its natural response to warding off this reaction in later life. The condition is not contagious, of course, but much like teething it can be a cause of regular sleepless nights for child and parent.

Just as in the other two definitions of an allergic response, atopic dermatitis sends the immune system into overdrive and causes chronic soreness and inflammation. Wherever there is an itch there is the desire to scratch and it is essential that you prevent this as much as possible. Rashes become much more sore and can begin to ooze when irritated further – but more than this, scratching will cause thickened skin tissue that results in dark, often unsightly patches and scars that might never disappear.

Most people will outgrow eczema: however, 15 million people in the UK[22] alone will live with the partial inability to ward off the plethora of irritants in the environment. As there are so many mast cells in the skin, given the sheer surface area, triggered histamine release can cause a severe urticarial reaction. Unlike other forms of eczema which we shall discuss shortly, atopic dermatitis outbreaks do not remain localised to the area of attack and can be widespread through the skin's surface.

These reactions come in response to both environmental triggers and – uniquely in the terms outlined so far – emotional triggers. Paul Herriot, Irish radio host for the station RTE, has spoken at length about stress around his working life being a key cause of 'flare-ups'. So intense were his outbreaks that his inability to avoid scratching left him lesions and scars across his body.[23]

The effect of stress on the body is not an exact science and is little understood in terms of true cause and effect. A contributing factor is undoubtedly the worry of actually having an outbreak – so the pragmatic steps are to understand the common triggers which you may encounter, leading to a calm approach based on fact and not fear. Self-help can be further improved by avoiding irritants as well – there are a host of products or environmental factors that spark overactive histamine release in the skin:

- **The obvious**
  Cigarette smoke
  Metals (especially nickel)
  Soaps, household cleaners and detergents
  Fabrics (wool and polyester are the main culprits)
  Fragrances in all forms
  Glues and adhesives

- **The less obvious**
  Antibacterial agents found in care products such as
      face and baby wipes
  Cocamidopropyl betaine which is used to thicken
      shampoos, soaps and lotions
  Para-phenylenediamine used in leather tanning
      and temporary tattoos

A common symptom of atopic dermatitis is the regular appearance of dry and scaly skin. This is a major problem, not just because of the discomfort experienced but because microscopic tears and cracks leave the protective layer open and even more susceptible to irritants and bacteria. It is essential to moisturise correctly as cracks and dryness on our outer surfaces firstly show a lack of retained water in the skin and leave it open to lose even more moisture over time. This can become a vicious circle.

Contact Dermatitis

As you might expect, contact dermatitis is far more common than its atopic counterpart as it is not strictly an allergy and accounts for 80–90 per cent of all cases.[24] The jargon tells us that it is a type 4 hypersensitivity reaction, which means it is a direct T lymphocyte effect. Put more simply, an irritant causes physical damage to the skin similar to serious abrasion or burns while an allergen triggers an immune response and causes a skin reaction.

Even though the immune trigger response is biologically different the triggers themselves are almost identical and the symptoms can be just as debilitating. Classic contact dermatitis agents are nickel (in watches and jewellery), gold and chromium.

Irritant Dermatitis

We also see a number of cases where harsh alkaline soaps, detergents and cleaning products have a major physical impact on the skin's surface. It is unsurprising that the classic irritants to avoid are:

- **The obvious**
  Industrial chemicals
  Solvents
  Skincare products containing alcohol
  Soaps and fragrances
  Bleach
  Wool
  Detergents

- **The less obvious**
  Paint
  Acidic foods
  Astringents

Interaction with any one of these will cause more localised damage versus an allergic reaction. As is the case with metallic irritants, the symptoms will only appear in the area affected, say on the wrist on the underside of one's watch in nickel contact dermatitis, or on the palms and fingers from an industrial worker using solvents etc. in irritant dermatitis. The output is very similar though and sufferers will have to bear redness, rashes and blistering as well as some burning and, often, swelling.

Diagnose, Avoid and Remedy

Diagnose

The way to diagnose contact and irritant dermatitis is usually to ask a few questions – has there been a change in the washing powder or soap the patient uses, for example? All cosmetics should be understood and considered, especially if the reaction is on the face. Hand dermatitis may be linked to occupation, such as the use of solvents.

Avoid

Avoidance for contact allergy and dermatitis is really about those steps you can take every day to ensure that your skin is in the best possible condition to limit the frequency of outbreaks and minimise the severity.

- *Go nuts for nuts*

    Water retention on the skin's surface is absolutely essential in repairing those micro tears and lesions discussed above, which leave serious gaps in the body's defence against irritants. Diet is key to ensuring a high intake of foods which promote skin water retention. The first thing to do, obviously, is to drink water in large quantities.

You might think you do this already – you don't. Two litres of water extra per day, on top of other drinks, should be considered a minimum. Try keeping bottles in the fridge, as we tend to opt for cold drinks – so having a regular supply of ice cold water to hand will make it more likely for you to choose this rather than soft drinks and sodas. As a snack eat a handful of nuts and cucumber sticks daily – they are great for you but also help maximise the plump youthful feeling on the skin you need. Finally, foods rich in omega-3 are fantastic as they are able to manage and rebalance the skin's oil production and give a significant immune boost when part of a regular weekly diet. Of course, you could opt for supplements, but don't! Processed versions will never replace the nutrients gleaned at the source – so eat whole, natural, high omega-3 foods like oily fish at least three times a week.

• Skin-drying drinks

No. Five cups of coffee a day does not count towards your water intake. Caffeinated drinks and alcohol constrict the blood vessels, which limits the nutrients that can be absorbed from all those good foods listed above. Furthermore both caffeine and alcohol are diuretics – they will actively dry you out. As extreme as cutting out caffeine and alcohol seems, it's surely a small price to pay for itch-free skin and great sleep.

• Heat exposure

Overly hot showers and sun exposure are something to be wary of when it comes to drying out the skin and also damaging it (often irreparably) at the same time. Even those without dermatitis will have felt the drying effects of a steaming hot shower and the heat rashes which result. Patients must avoid this. It puts the skin under completely avoidable strain and serves to reverse all the good work you have been doing in the preceding steps, by reopening and deepening tears on the skin's surface.

Sunbathing is similar, and a high-quality factor 30 (ideally 50) is a must for prolonged spells in even mild temperatures. A bigger concern is the wind exposure we experience often unknowingly while at the beach or in the great outdoors. Wind dries out the skin very quickly and then leaves you open to the elements for the rest of the day. Plan ahead. Again factor 50 will keep the skin moisturised in the toughest winds but also rubbing Vaseline on your lips or using a salve of choice on and into the corners of the lips and around the base of the nostrils will have huge preventative power.

- ***Ensure restful sleep***

We know what you are thinking. It is easy for us to say when we aren't awake all night, itching to the point of tears. But follow the points above and not only will your symptoms reduce significantly but so will the frequency of your episodes. Sleep is the true fountain of youth and health and following the process above to only get two more hours' deep sleep will have monumental effects on your body's ability to heal.

Remedy

Navigating the ladder of intervention means a process of trialling what works best for you. The best way to do this is to start at the first step and move down. You might find that one step gives you the best relief or maybe it is one or more used in combination. Before undergoing the process do make sure you are in consultation with your GP.

Ladder of intervention

1 Emollients

2 Steroid creams

3 Wraps

• *Emollients*

Emollients are ways of soothing the skin, just by hydrating and protecting it. Ointments, creams and lotions are three different examples of emollients. Ointments are thick and unsightly, but stick well to skin and eczema, so are great for use at night when they can be plastered all over the body, not just on the eczema areas. Creams are thinner and are absorbed more quickly, so are good for use during the day. Lotions aren't really effective in this situation as they dry out too quickly, but they can be helpful in hair-bearing areas.

• *Steroid creams*

Steroid creams can also be used in combination with emollients – wait until the ointments etc. have been absorbed and the skin is fairly smooth. Fingertip units are how we measure the amount of steroid cream or ointment to be applied, as per the table on the next page.

Always use steroid creams or ointments under the supervision of your doctor. The general rule is to use milder steroid creams first, then work up to stronger ones if required.

Hydrocortisone 0.1 per cent is the mildest and this can be progressed up to 2.5 per cent. From there Betamethasone 0.025 per cent progressed up to 0.1 per cent and finally Clobetasol 0.05 per cent.

Fingertip units

Age	Face & Neck	1 Arm & Hand	1 Leg & Foot	Trunk (front)	Trunk (back) including buttocks
3–6 months	1	1	1.5	1	1.5
1–2 years	1.5	1.5	2	2	3
3–5 years	1.5	2	3	3	3.5
6–10 years	2	2.5	4.5	3.5	5
10+ – adults	2.5	4	8	7	8

• *Wraps*

Wraps can also be effective in treating eczema. They are basically wet bandages that are wrapped around affected areas, helping to keep the area moist and cool. They are also useful in protecting eczematous areas from scratching. The routine can be quite time-consuming but it is well worth it. The process takes 2–3 days and once it is complete you will want to ensure you are regularly moisturising the skin daily thereafter.

How to wrap and seal

1.   Leave some bandages to soak in a clean bowl of water.

2.   Bathe the body or just the affected area in lukewarm water for 20 minutes. Ensure the bath is clean and that no soap is used.

3.   Pat your skin dry with a fresh clean towel, laundered with non-bio washing formula.

4.   Apply a layer of simple aqueous or natural eczema cream to the affected area(s).

5.   Wring out the bandages, removing all excess liquid. The bandages should be damp – NOT soaking wet.

6.   Wrap the bandages over the moisturised skin and cover with a dry layer. Tracksuit bottoms are ideal for the lower body and a clean close-fitting sweatshirt for the upper body.

7.   Keep the wraps on for at least three hours or until they are no longer damp to the touch. It's absolutely fine to keep them on overnight.

8.   Repeat this process twice a day if you can, although we understand that damp bandages under clothing while at school or at work might be uncomfortable. We would suggest starting the process on a Friday and following the steps over the course of the weekend to avoid discomfort out of the house.

9.   By Monday morning your skin will have reached the optimised moisture level. Maintain this by referring back to the avoidance techniques above (especially the 'Heat exposure' section) and in consultation with your GP continue applying a daily moisturiser to the whole body.

In Summary

Contact allergies are often those that people (especially young people) are most fearful of, given the very physical appearance of reactions on the face, hands and body. For sufferers the story stretches far beyond this, as rather than manageable seasonal outbreaks the reality can be year-long management of discomfort of the body and mind.

6.

Anaphylaxis

The Statistics

Death from anaphylaxis is every allergic patient or parent's greatest worry. The actual incidence of death from food allergy anaphylaxis is around three per million food allergy sufferers of age 0–19 years (not the general population) per year. It is even lower for adults. You are less likely to be a food allergy sufferer and die of anaphylaxis than to be a member of the general population and be murdered. Only six people a year die of food anaphylaxis in the UK.

It is rare – but it *does* happen. The art is to properly identify those with true food allergy by using blood and skin prick testing, and train them and those around them regarding avoidance and use of adrenaline injections when indicated. There should be no reluctance among true allergy sufferers to use injectable adrenaline when it is available and required. Failure to use it in a true anaphylaxis situation can lead to death. There is virtually no risk from one or two uses of emergency adrenaline injectors – such as EpiPen. Over ten EpiPen injections would have to be given before a toxic level of adrenaline was reached.

Using an EpiPen (or equivalent)

An EpiPen is a disposable, pre-filled, automated injection device that administers adrenaline (or epinephrine – it's the same) in the event of severe allergic reaction.[25] In most cases you will have been prescribed an EpiPen and will know that you should carry it at all times and use it at the first signs of any symptom.

In the event that you are helping someone who is having a severe allergic reaction then the protocol is as follows:

1. Have a friend or neighbour call an ambulance immediately or if you are alone use the EpiPen first!
2. Find the patient's EpiPen, which is a board marker-sized bright orange cylinder with a blue cap on one end.
3. Hold the pen in a pistol grip with the blue cap pointing upwards towards you and pull the blue cap off by pulling upwards – do not bend or twist.
4. The pen is now ready to be used. Swing and press the orange end into the patient's mid-outer thigh until you hear a 'click'. Hold it tight for ten seconds.
5. If you were alone now call the emergency services.

Frequently Asked Questions

Why do bee or wasp stings sometimes cause anaphylaxis?

Venom from these stings sets up an immune reaction, so the first time you are stung anaphylaxis doesn't happen, unless you have a genetic predisposition to this – which is not possible to test for and can only be guessed at. It is the subsequent sting(s) which cause the problem. Furthermore, the venom causes vasodilation – the opening up of blood vessels around the sting site. This means that quickly after being stung the venom is circulating around the body, interacting with IgE and causing mast cell degranulation very widely, with resultant anaphylaxis.

Are there any treatments for food allergy?

Currently, avoiding the food you are allergic to is the only way to protect against a reaction. There are some desensitisation therapies being investigated, but none is available yet. Standard anti-allergy treatment such as antihistamines, antileukotrienes and steroids can help in acute exacerbations.

Does eating peanuts during pregnancy lower the risk of peanut allergies/intolerance for the child?

No, it is part of the development of the immune system, which occurs after birth, that leads to allergy.

Are allergies on the increase?

Yes, recent statistics show that the prevalence of allergy is rising at an alarming rate, particularly in the Western world.

Are intolerances on the increase?

They appear to be, although data is sparse. It may be due to easier access to information – Dr Google.

Do food allergens remain on objects like a mobile phone or a keyboard?

Yes, food allergens can potentially remain on objects if they are not carefully cleaned. However, simply touching an object that contains something you are allergic to would either do nothing or at worst possibly cause a rash on your skin at the site of contact. Without swallowing any of the allergen, it's highly unlikely you would have any further reaction. It is a common myth that you can have a severe reaction from simply touching something without eating the food. Many studies have shown that if you wash your hands well with soap and water, as well as thoroughly clean the contaminated surface with detergent, you can effectively remove the allergen.

Note: Gel-based alcohol hand cleaners will *not* remove allergens from your skin: soap and water is best.

Can food allergies develop in an adult?

Although most food allergies develop when you are a child, they can, in rare cases, develop when you are an adult. The most common food allergies for adults are shellfish – both crustaceans and molluscs – as well as tree nuts, peanuts (groundnuts) and fish. Most adults with food allergies have had their allergy since they were children. An allergic reaction to a food can sometimes be missed in an adult because symptoms such as vomiting or diarrhoea can be mistaken for flu or food poisoning. Adults don't always pay close attention to symptoms, which can be dangerous since crucial hints can be missed and place the adult at risk if they continue to eat the food.

What is oral allergy syndrome?

Oral allergy syndrome is something that can develop in adulthood. Also known as pollen-food syndrome, it is caused by cross-reacting allergens found in pollen and raw fruits, vegetables and some tree nuts. This is not a food allergy, though the symptoms occur after eating food, which can be confusing. Rather, this is a pollen allergy. The symptoms of oral allergy syndrome are an itchy mouth or tongue, or swelling of the lips or tongue. Classic oral allergy syndrome occurs in birch tree pollen allergy and eating foods with an antigen structure very similar to the birch Bet vi: namely apple, hazelnut, carrot, cherry, pear, tomato, celery, potato and peach. The lip and mouth swelling can be mistaken for anaphylaxis and can be the cause of anxiety and ambulance call-outs.

What are the chances of having a severe reaction to airborne food allergens?

Virtually none. No study has ever conclusively proven that allergens become airborne and cause symptoms to develop. Those with food allergies only have severe reactions after eating the allergic food. Many people with peanut allergy also worry about the dust from peanuts, particularly on aeroplanes. Most reactions probably happen after touching and ingesting peanut dust that may be on tray tables or other surfaces. Surface contact does not cause anaphylaxis.

Can you grow out of food allergies?

Yes. This is an important point to emphasise. Children generally, but not always, outgrow allergies to milk, eggs, soy and wheat. New research indicates that up to 25 per cent of children may outgrow their peanut allergy, with slightly fewer expected to outgrow a tree nut allergy. There is no need to assume your child's food allergy will be lifelong, though for some this may be the case. If you develop food allergy as an adult, the chances are much lower that you will outgrow it. Food allergies in adults tend to be lifelong, though there has not been a lot of research in this area.

How much does it cost to get tested for food allergies?

This varies worldwide, of course. In the UK, a standard blood allergy screening test costs from £250–£500, depending on where you are having it done. Skin prick tests usually cost around £15 per agent tested – so the price varies depending on how many antigens you have tested.

What is gluten? How common is gluten allergy?

Gluten is a protein found in grains, such as wheat, barley and rye. Some people are allergic to wheat, but that is not the same as a gluten allergy. Gluten allergy is a misleading term commonly confused with wheat allergy. There is no such thing as a gluten allergy, but there is a condition called coeliac disease. This is an intolerance to gluten, not an allergy.

What is the difference between allergy and immunity to infection?

Little really: the recognition process is very similar, though the site of action differs, and the antibodies used to mediate the reaction differ, as does the end effect – allergy ends in mast cell degranulation, immunity in pathogen destruction. As we have discussed, the body's natural surveillance system is on a constant lookout for any noxious or infectious agents it may encounter and is ready to repel them – the classic type I hypersensitivity allergic response with IgE. It's rather like a military early warning radar against enemy aeroplanes. But when these surveillance systems in the body fail to neutralise an unwanted agent, consequences occur – we get partially poisoned, or a parasite lodges or we catch a cold, etc. But with a virus type of infection, a healthy system is able to resolve the problem by itself within a few days of launching a different immune response (IgM and IgG), where antibodies are quickly made *de novo*, without any prior recognition. In the military analogy, if the early warning system fails due to Stealth (?!), quickly adapt and learn how to strike before it kills you.

With immunity to infection, as in allergy, antibodies are pre-made ready for immediate action, because of prior recognition – you can't catch the same virus twice for the same reason, as you have memory cells, just as you do in allergy.

Conclusion

The big messages of this book are:

- Take allergy seriously
- Closely analyse your symptoms and life so that you can be accurately tested if you believe you have an allergy
- Consult your doctor
- Understand the difference between allergy and intolerance
- Read this book carefully and consult with your doctor

How to help yourself:

- Diagnose
- Avoid
- Remedy

References

1. www.telegraph.co.uk/news/2017/06/09/red-velvet-cupcakes-fuelling-rise-allergies-dietician-says/

2. Igea, J. M.: 'The history of the idea of allergy', *Allergy* (2013) 68: 966–73, p. 966

3. Turner, P. J., Gowland, M. H., Sharma, V., Ierodiakonou, D., Harper, N., Garcez, T., ... Boyle, R. J.: 'Increase in anaphylaxis-related hospitalizations but no increase in fatalities: An analysis of United Kingdom national anaphylaxis data, 1992-2012' *The Journal of Allergy and Clinical Immunology* (2015) 135: 956–963.

4. www.aaaai.org/about-aaaai/newsroom/allergy-statistics

5. www.goodtherapy.org/blog/stress-anxiety-food-allergies-1107127

6. my.clevelandclinic.org/health/articles/milk-allergies

7. AAW 2016 FSA: www.food.gov.uk/allergen-resources

8. www.healthline.com/health/allergies/ingested-contact-inhaled

9. www.allergywatch.org/basic/airborne_allergens.pdf

10. ophthalmologytimes.modernmedicine.com/ophthalmology times/news/managing-treatment-options-atopic-kerato conjunctivitis

11. www.rac.co.uk/drive/advice/road-safety/hay-fever-a-hazard-for-motorists/

12. www.allergy-clinic.co.uk/allergies/airway-allergy/hayfever/

13. www.channelnewsasia.com/news/lifestyle/yes-you-can-develop-food-allergies-as-an-adult-9122226

14. www.netdoctor.co.uk/conditions/allergy-and-asthma/a6102/food-allergy

15. www.aaaai.org/conditions-and-treatments/library/allergy-library/food-allergy

16. Hertzler, S. R., Huynh, B. C., Savaiano, D. A.: 'How much lactose is low lactose?', *Journal of the American Dietetic Association* (1996) 96: 243–46

17. www.camnutri.com/histamine-intolerance-p-90.html?detail=7&cPath=22

18. www.foodsmatter.com/allergy_intolerance/food_intolerance/articles/hunter_huntley_food_intol.html

19. www.panic-attacks.co.uk/course/4-panic-attack-symptoms-hyperventilation-over-breathing/

20. nationaleczema.org/eczema/types-of-eczema/

21. www.babycenter.com/0_eczema-in-babies_10872.bc

22. www.allergyuk.org/about/latest-news/310-eczema-are-we-just-scratching-the-surface

23. www.independent.ie/life/health-wellbeing/health-features/rte-radio-presenter-on-his-battle-with-eczema-i-had-lesions-and-scratch-marks-36125185.html

24. www.pharmacytimes.com/publications/issue/2013/april2013/treatment-and-management-of-dermatitis

25. www.epipen.ca/en/about-epipen/how-to-use